Letter from the Publisher

Amanda Klenner

Sage is one of those herbs that just about everyone knows. To some, the thought of sage brings the smell of a delicious herb used to spice some wonderfully starchy foods or meats as a savory delight. Indeed, this delicious herb is a wonderful carminative, easing the digestion of heavy meals as well as adding a wonderful flavor. Others remember being given sage tea with some honey as a child when they had a cough. The aromatic tea is a beautiful way to enjoy the healing benefits of sage. Others may think of sage wisdom, something elders have learned from years of experience through hard work, dedication, remorse, and doubt. This wisdom gained through the years and passed on is thought of as sage; well-seasoned. Interestingly enough, sage has even been used to increase cognitive abilities of the elderly who suffer from dementia and Alzheimer's.

One of the things I love about sage is that it is an herb that is widely found in most kitchens and gardens. Plants in the *salvia* genus are almost everywhere and can be found in the wild in many different climates, making it a widely accessible herb. Indeed it is an herb for "the people." Most herbs have a tendency to be either warm or cool, hot or cold. However, sage is interesting in the way that different people experience its energetics differently. To some, chewing on a sage leaf cools the mouth, while to others it is warming. It is often used in menopause to treat the all too common night sweats. This is a great example of how sage can be cooling to the body. When a person has a cold and drinks warm sage tea (or another herbal tea with sage honey) it can have a warming effect on the body. Just another example of how sage works so well for most, no matter what their body type or constitution.

So how does sage work for you? Chew on a leaf and see if your mouth feels warm or cool. Drink some warm tea and take note of how your body feels. Now try some cool tea. How does that feel? What about sage honey? How do you feel that working in your body?

Sage is a wonderful herb to experiment with and to really build the ability to greatly appreciate and understand an herb. I challenge you to go online or find a good plant identification book and see if you can find the local *Salvia* that grows around you. If your local salvia is safe, see how that works compared to *Salvia officinalis* and take the time to sit down and build a relationship with this wise herbal ally.

Green Blessings,

- *Amanda*

Table of Contents

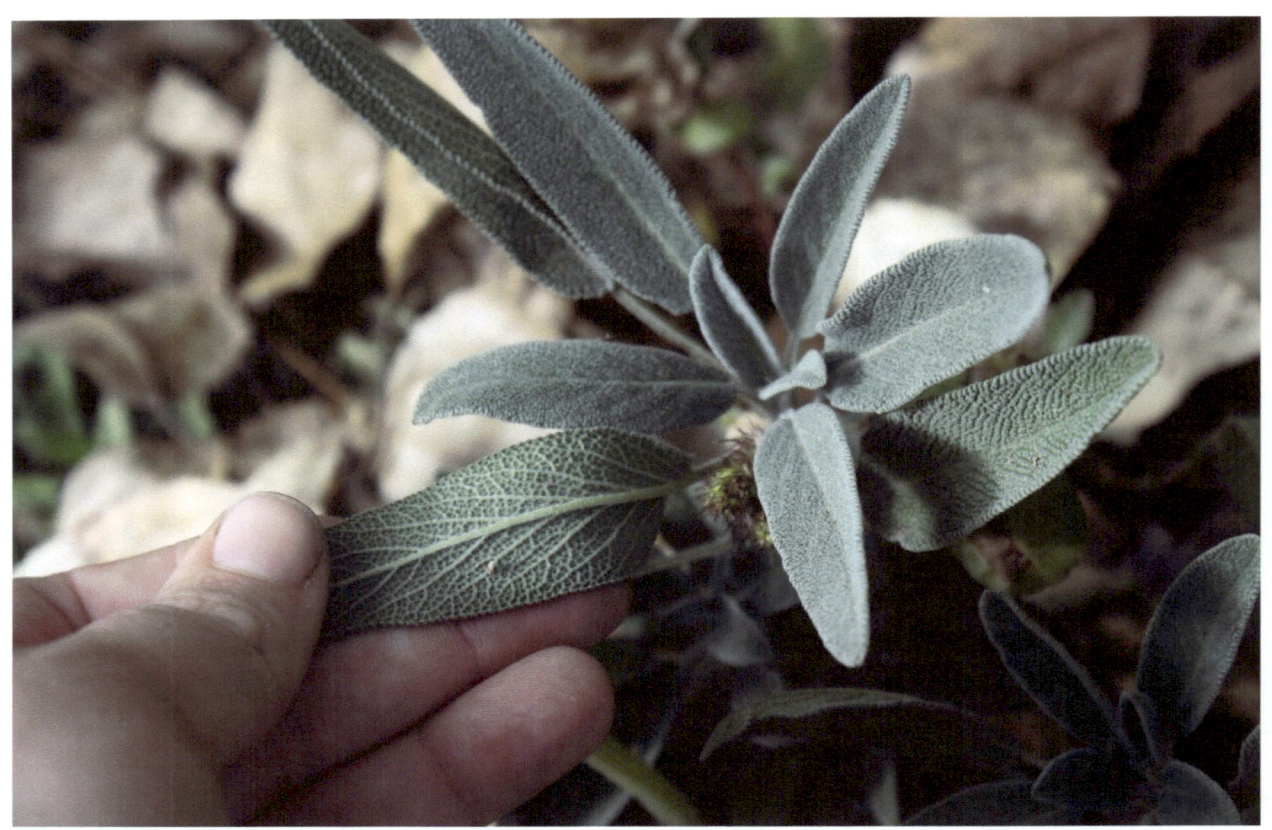

Sage Herbal Monograph

Angela Justis

Common Name: sage, garden sage, common sage, culinary sage

Latin Name: *Salvia officinalis, Salvia spp., S. sclarea, S. verbenaca, S. apiana, S. subincisa, S. carnosa*

Family: Lamiaceae

ACTIONS:

astringent, antibacterial, antifungal, antiseptic, anti-catarrhal, antihidrotic, carminative, emmenagogue, febrifuge, nervine, spasmolytic, stimulant

DESCRIPTION:

As member of the Lamiaceae (mint) family, sage has the common Lamiaceae characteristics of a square stem and opposite leaves. The leaves of the common or garden sage are wrinkly with an oblong shape and a light silvery, green color. If gently rubbed, sage will give off it's delightful, characteristic scent. The flowers are borne on spikes and have the typical Lamiaceae appearance with the petals forming lips; two fused petals on top and 3 fused petals on the bottom. Flower color can vary but is often a lovely blue-lavender. Comprised of many different varieties of plants with just as many variations in appearance, sage is a wonderful group of plants that offers great healing and support to us. This lovely genus of plants can be used interchangeably, with certain members of the genus offering their own particular healing strengths.

Long used as a healing remedy, the *officinalis* part of sage's name indicates its classification as a plant that is used in medicine, and it has been used as such throughout history. Furthermore, *Salvia* comes from the word salvare, which means to save or heal, so it is no surprise that sage has long been recognized as a revitalizing tonic that strengthens the body, mind, and spirit.

Sage has an interesting ability to be either warming or cooling depending on the person. It is also a drying herb, which is a wonderful remedy for inflammation of the mouth, throat, and upper respiratory tract. It soothes the mucous membranes while reducing phlegm and acting as an antimicrobial to help relieve infections. Use as a gargle for afflictions of the mouth and throat including laryngitis, pharyngitis, tonsillitis, and gum disease. Particularly, it will alleviate the pain of canker sores with repeated applications as a mouthwash.[1] It is excellent for cold and flus when there is an overproduction of irritating mucus, and is especially helpful when taken at the first sign of illness. Sage also helps to stop excessive, debilitating sweating during prolonged illness.

It is rich in volitile oils that help to stimulate digestion, easing indigestion where there is gas. It can relieve cramping and bloating, and aid in the digestion of food, particularly meals of heavy, fatty dishes. The astringent property helps to arrest diarrhea.

Sage is an amazing remedy for women. It is an emmenagogue, which can be used for suppressed and irregular menstruation. It can also act as an aid for easing cramping, heavy bleeding, and even flooding during menopause. Sage is well known for it's ability to dry up breast milk and can help during weaning or to curb excessive flow. Rosemary Gladstar uses sage as a compress for mastitis because she explains that sage "takes the pressure off

---

[1] DIY Herbs- Sage

the breasts."[1] For these same reasons, sage should be avoided during pregnancy and breast feeding. Sage is wonderful for women going through menopause. It helps to calm anxiety and insomnia and alleviates irregular menstruation that can accompany menopause. It is specific for hot flashes during menopause that cause heavy sweating. It also "clearly promotes estrogen production, and may lower FSH and LH surges during the menopausal years."[2]

This silver beauty is a profound, grounding nervine that is often overlooked, and indeed can help to restore the mind and the nervous system. It is grounding and centering, relieving nervousness and anxiety, depression, and exhaustion while aiding memory. In fact, Kiva Rose states that sage is "more than a nervine, this is a tonic for rebuilding the nervous system where there has been deep and long lasting trauma. Specifically useful where there's shaking and tremors, anxiety with overwhelming fear, and profound burnout."[3]

Sage can benefit those who are aging and need to restore health and vitality. The very word "sage" brings to mind the wisdom of age, which is the wisdom of the sage or wise person. It is reputed by herbalists to slow the aging process while bestowing vitality to the sage elder. According to Susun Weed, not only is sage full of vitamins and minerals, it is "filled with antioxidants that retard wrinkles and grey hair and help prevent cancer [while providing] heart-healthy oils."[4] Matthew Wood goes on to explain that sage is a wonderful herb for those going through the change of life, be they women or men, when hormonal production shifts from the ovaries and testes to the adrenal glands.[5] Interestingly, sage may be helpful for our wise elders as a memory aid. David Hoffman explains that research has found that sage tea inhibits acetylcholinesterase, the enzyme that breaks down acetylcholine. This breakdown contributes to short-term memory loss sometime experienced as senile dementia by some elders.[6]

---

[1] Rosemary Gladstar's Garden Wisdoms: Sage and Thyme
[2] Menopausal Years,pg 48
[3] A Few of my Favorite Calming & Uplifting Herbs

[4] Menopausal Years,112
[5] DIY Herbs- Sage
[6] DIY Herbs- Sage

Sage can work well as a topical remedy to reduce inflammation and swelling. Due to it's high antimicrobial essential oil content it is wonderful for cleansing and soothing skin issues. Use it on abrasions, burns, and ulcerated conditions to cleanse and dry up secretions. It also makes a great poultice or can be soaked for inflamed, painful joints and muscles.

Preparations and Dosage

Infusion: Steep 1 to 2 teaspoons of dried leaves in 1 cup of water for up to 10 minutes. Drink this three times per day. Sage infusion is particularly lovely with lemon and honey for throat issues. Rosemary Gladstar combines sage with rosemary and thyme to brew up a very emotionally grounding tea.[1]

Tincture Take 10 to 40 drops up to 4 times per day during acute situations. Otherwise, enjoy 1 to 3 times per week.

Sage can also be cooked into your food or infused into honey and vinegar to enjoy.

Safety Considerations

Aptly said by David Hoffman, "any herb that is used as a flavor in cooking, you can assume a fair degree of safety and lack of toxicity."[2] However, because of it's emmenagogue action and ability to dry breast milk, do not use sage if pregnant or nursing. Also due to its astringent nature, please watch for any excess dryness while using sage and either stop its usage or combine with moistening, mucilaginous herbs such as marshmallow or licorice. Due to the high essential oil content, sage should not be consumed for long periods of time as the oils can build up in the liver and kidneys. *Salvias* can, for the most part, be used interchangeably, but be sure to check before using them in this way, however please don't confuse them with plants in the *Artemisias* genus such as woodworm, sagebrush, and mugwort.

---

[1] Rosemary Gladstar's Garden Wisdoms: Sage and Thyme
[2] Rosemary Gladstar's Garden Wisdoms: Sage and Thyme

References

Books

1. Grieve, Mrs. M., A Modern Herbal, Random House, 1973
2. Hoffman, David, The Complete Illustrated Herbal,
3. Element Books, 1996
4. McIntyre, Anne, Flower Power, Henry Holt & Company, Inc., 1996
5. Tilgner, Sharol, N.D., Herbal Medicine from the Heart of the Earth, Wise Acres Press, Inc., 1999
6. Trickey, Ruth, Women, Hormones & The Menstrual Cycle,
7. Allen & Unwin, 1998
8. Weed, Susun S., Menopausal Years The Wise Woman Way,
9. Ash Tree Publishing, 1992

Websites

- Rosemary Gladstar's Garden Wisdoms: Sage and Thyme: https://www.youtube.com/watch?v=gO89--te8F4&feature=youtu.be
- DIY Herbs- Sage:
- https://www.youtube.com/watch?v=Pvm1t3eI_As
- A Few of my Favorite Calming & Uplifting Herbs:
- http://bearmedicineherbals.com/a-few-of-my-favorite-calming-uplifting-herbs.html
- Salvia: A Plant Teacher for Grounding & Presence:
- http://bearmedicineherbals.com/salvia-a-plant-teacher-for-grounding-presence.html

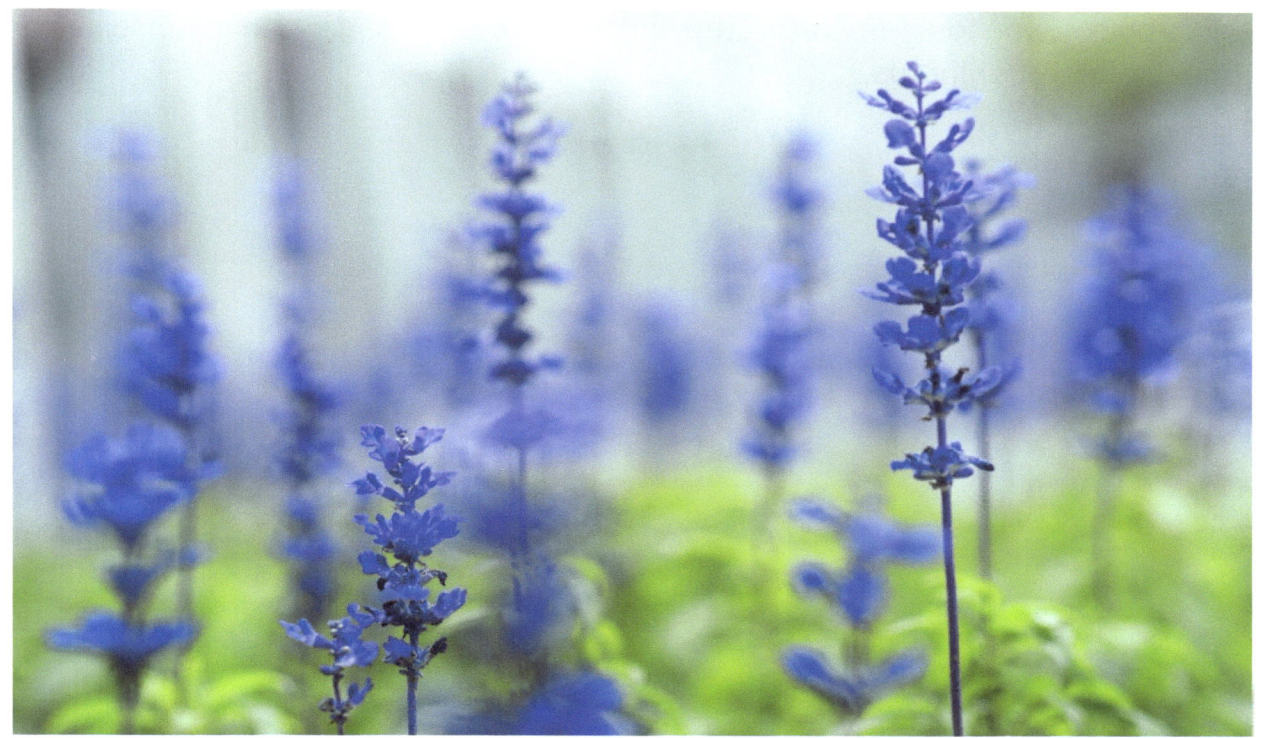

Sage Flower Essence

Charis Denny

We cannot all be the wizened, old sage up on the mountaintop, living alone and dispensing wisdom and knowledge to those brave enough to make the arduous journey to our hidden lair – nor would we all want to! What we can do is utilize sage flower essence as our own expert advisor concerning the meanings of our life experiences.

In a perfect world, we would move through the trials and tribulations of life always catching on to and internalizing the lessons they provide to us. Unfortunately, though, sometimes we fail to have the ability to perceive the higher purpose and meanings in life's challenges. This can lead us to a feeling that we have been ill-treated or even victimized.

Sage flower essence helps us age and mature in a healthy manner, learning to distill our negative experiences in such a way that we are able to glean from them authentic wisdom. By doing this, we enhance our capacity to experience a deep and healing inner peace. As sage is especially indicated for reflecting upon our life experiences as we age, it is ideal for helping us think back upon our life and step into the role of sage and counselor for those coming behind us.

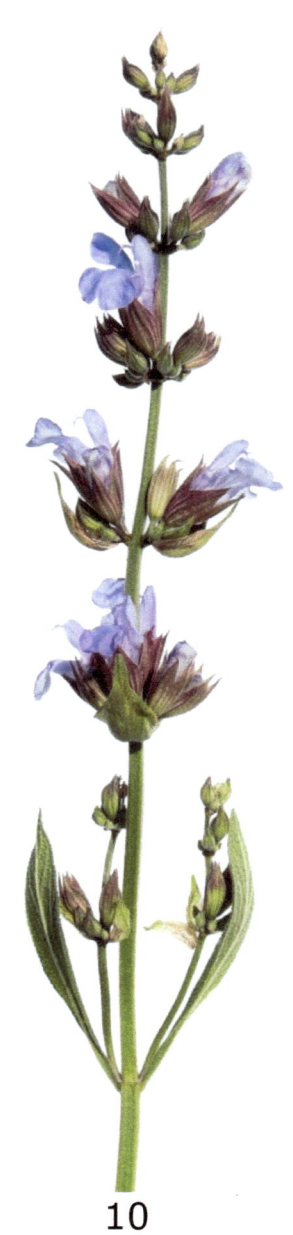

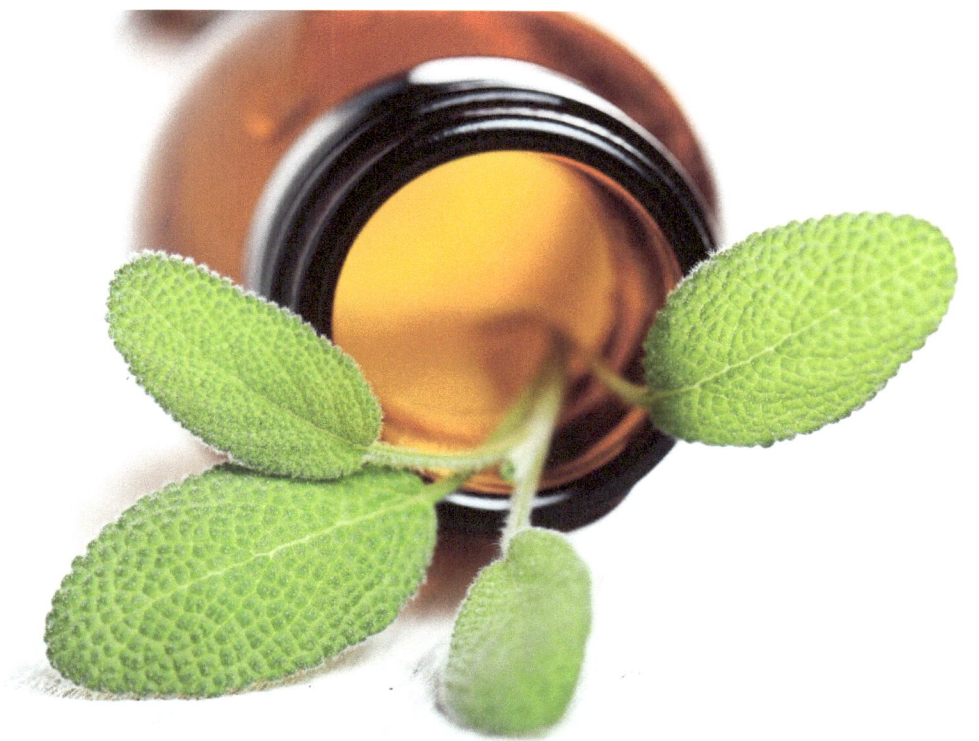

Sage Essential Oil Profile

Lea Harris

Sage, or Dalmatian sage, essential oil is distilled from the dried leaves of the *Salvia officinalis* plant.

Safety Information

Before we delve into the therapeutic properties of sage, it's important to look at the safety information. Sage is a good example of not assuming the essential oil is safe just because the herb may be.

Sage essential oil should never be taken orally. If used topically, sage essential oil should not be used at more than a 0.4% dilution (two drops of essential oil in a teaspoon of carrier oil is 0.5%) due to thujone content. If you are prone to seizures, are pregnant, or are breastfeeding, it is recommended you avoid this oil altogether.

Other types of sage essential oil that are not hazardous but may have some concerns:

- Greek Sage (*Salvia fruticosa/Salvia triloba*) – avoid using around children under age 10 due to 1,8-cineole content (can cause slowed respiration)
- Spanish Sage (*Salvia lavandulifolia/Salvia hispanorum*) – avoid if pregnant or breastfeeding due to abortifacient properties
- White Sage (*Salvia apiana*) - avoid using on/around children under age 10 due to 1,8-cineole content (can cause slowed respiration)
- Wild Mountain Sage (*Hemizygia petiolata*) – avoid using on/around children under age 2; moderate risk of irritation and skin sensitization; drug interaction (drugs metabolized by CYP2D6).

Sage essential oils that are not known to be hazardous are:

- African Wild Sage (*Tarchonanthus camphoratus*)
- Blue Mountain Sage (*Salvia stenophylla*)

Now that we know the safety parameters, let's take a look at sage's therapeutic properties.

Therapeutic Properties

- Anti-inflammatory – added to a lotion can relieve rheumatism and arthritis
- Anti-bacterial – used in a tooth cleanser can be helpful against periodontal disease
- Anti-septic & Astringent – when used in a facial wash, can help clear up acne, dermatitis, and eczema
- Anti-spasmodic – can help relieve menstrual cramps
- Digestive – inhaling or massaging over the abdomen can strengthen digestion and increase appetite
- Expectorant – breaks up congestion when inhaled, diffused, or used in a steam inhalation
- Regenerative – can be added to shampoo to treat alopecia and dandruff

Although essential oils do not contain hormones, some of them, like sage essential oil, can imitate estrogen. The benefits of this include the regulation of the menstrual cycle (treating delayed menstruation, scanty menstruation, or no menstruation), cramping, sweating, or other PMS symptoms. It is also useful to relieve painful menstruation when used in moderation.

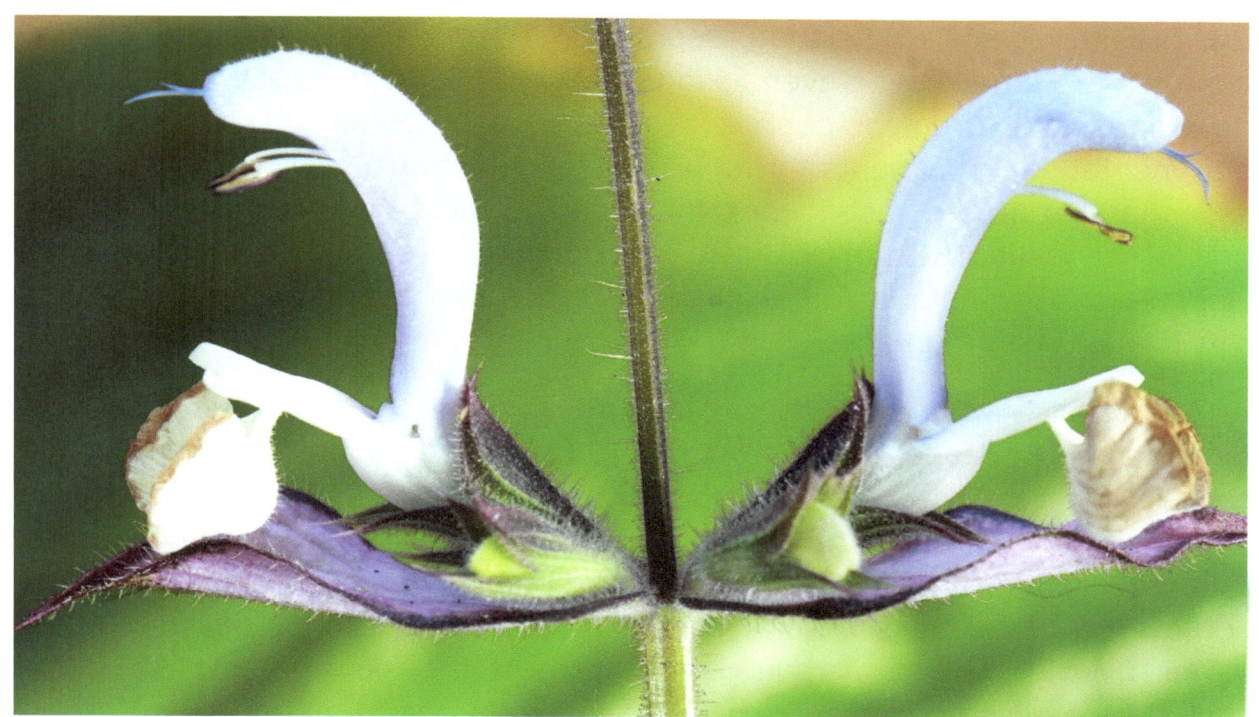

Clary Sage Essential Oil

Cassie Soule

Salvia sclarea is an amazing essential oil in the Lamiaceae family and is occasionally considered a bit controversial. This is the same family as *Lavender officinalis*, and it has many of the same calming and sedative type qualities.

Essential oils can be found in different parts of a plant, but clary sage essential oil is distilled from the leaves and the flowers. The scent of clary sage can be described as herbaceous, yet sweet. It's been interesting to hear people talk about their immediate reactions to the aroma of clary sage. Sometimes they love it and sometimes they hate it, but the really fascinating part is that many grow to love it or even crave it, even if they initially did not care for it. This is the power of this little essential oil.

According to Sue Clark in her book Essential Chemistry for Aromatherapy, clary sage can have "powerful euphoric effects."[1] She also lists a variety of therapeutic uses like treating depression, lifting the spirit, and use for creativity. Some have even suggested that *Salvia sclarea* should be developed as a drug for depression.[1] Because of its benefits for emotional and mental health benefits through its calming actions, clary sage, like many essential oils, is best used when inhaled. The most common use is for PMS and other issues with the female reproductive system. Some people find clary sage very helpful for respiratory issues like asthma and coughs, but this is a less common use.

As an herbalist and aromatherapy educator I can tell you many stories of the benefits of clary sage, especially for PMS pains and emotions. Often, women can simply open the bottle and breathe it in to find immediate relief from cramping and irritability. I have also heard from clients who have wanted quick relief and simply dropped the oil directly on their stomachs, though some found it to be slightly irritating to the skin. This particular reaction varies from person to person, but to protect the skin from irritation one should always use clary sage when it has been properly diluted.

Safety considerations

Mindy Green and Kathi Keville mention that *Salvia sclarea* essential oil contains a ketone "that mimics estrogen, so women who suffer from breast cysts and uterine fibroids or other estrogen related disorders should avoid long term use until more is understood about this action."[2]

The other safety consideration has to do with using clary sage during pregnancy. As a former doula and childbirth professional, this is a very important issue to me. Most midwives and doulas will tell you not to use it because it will stimulate uterine contractions. I've also heard highly revered people in the aromatherapy world say there is no concern with use during pregnancy because there is no evidence to back up this claim. When it comes to an essential oil that seems to have strong anecdotal safety concerns, we fall to what is called the precautionary principle, which is used

[1] Clark, Sue. Essential Chemistry for Aromatherapy.
[1] Rhind, Jennifer Peace.   Essential Oils A Handbook for Aromatherapy Practice
[2] Green, Mindy & Keville, Kathi. Aromatherapy A Complete Guide to the Healing Art

in the field of epidemiology. The precautionary principle basically explains that until standards are set for safety, it should not be used.

A couple of years ago I was holding a workshop for birth professionals on herbs and essential oils for pregnancy and birth. One of the midwives was pregnant, and she told me how just being in the room where a bottle of clary sage was used to stimulate a client's stalled labor also triggered her own contractions. Once she left the room, the contractions stopped. This is a very powerful reaction that is fairly common, although rarely reported. Again, here we see the strength of clary sage.

Practical application

Clary sage can be diluted and used in a relaxing bath, in a body or foot massage, or for a gentle belly massage to treat PMS discomfort. It can also be inhaled directly from the bottle, or used either on its own or in combination with other essential oils in a personal inhaler or diffuser. For added relaxing and calming benefits, *Salvia sclarea* blends nicely with other floral oils like lavender, chamomile, geranium, or rose.

Clary Sage Bath and Massage Oil

Ingredients

- 2 oz unscented vegetable oil (avocado, peach kernel, coconut, etc.)
- 12-15 drops *Salvia sclarea* (clary sage) essential oil

Directions

Combine ingredients in a glass bottle and shake gently. Use within 6-9 months and then discard. For a relaxing bath, add 1 teaspoon of the blend as needed. For a massage, use just enough to create a "slip" during a calming massage.

Diffusion Blend for Depression

For depression, clary sage blends well with citrus like bergamot or mandarin.

Ingredients

- 2 drops of *Salvia sclarea* (clary sage) essential oil
- 2 drops of mandarin (*Citrus reticulata*) essential oil
- 2 drops of lavender (*Lavender officinalis*) essential oil
- 3 drops of grapefruit (*Citrus paradisi*) essential oil

Directions

Add drops to a small essential oil bottle and gently shake. Add three drops of oil to a diffuser or simmering pot of water for 30 minutes, 2-3 times a day as needed.

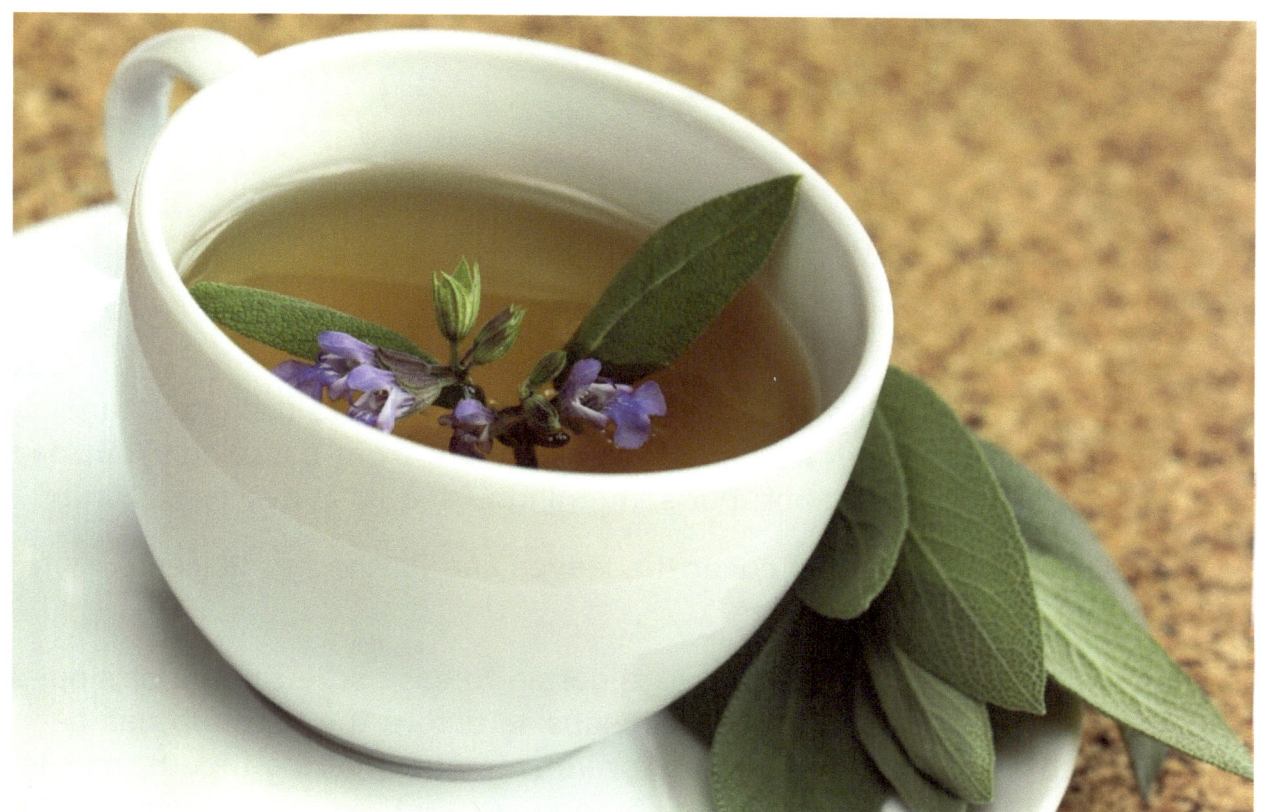

Sage Tea

Carol Little

Do you have a signal that tells you that your body is fighting something? Many folks develop a sudden headache. Others, a raspy cough. My own telltale sign is sudden tenderness in my throat; that scratchy, little catch in the throat that often quickly becomes akin to razor-sharp pain, signaling the possible arrival of a new invader.

My go-to herbal remedy in this situation? Garden sage (*Salvia officinalis*).

Herbal remedies take many forms. In this case, it's a tea, infusion, or tisane. Really, it's all the same thing. Hot water causes the sage leaves to offer the gift of healing to your sore throat!

Sage Infusion

Ingredients

- 1-2 oz sage leaves, fresh or dried (pro tip, roughly 8-10 leaves)
- boiling water

Directions

Place your sage leaves into a 1-quart canning jar. I like to use glass canning jars with lids to keep the aromatic, healing steam from escaping. You may also use a cup, mug, or teapot, but something with a lid is best.

Pour enough boiling water to cover the leaves and fill the jar. Place lid on jar and let steep for 10 -15 minutes.

The resulting infusion can be used as a gargle to ease sore throats or sipped as a soothing tea. Often, the pain will subside before the first cup has been finished! Medicinally, this tea is used for inflammations of the mouth, tonsils, and throat because the mucous membranes are soothed by the volatile oils. The therapeutic dose is 3-4 cups of sage tea per day, and definitely gargle or roll the warm tea around in your mouth, allowing it to reach the back of your throat before swallowing.

If you're a gardener, you may already have sage on hand. I have harvested it year round, but I snip leaves throughout the summer and autumn to ensure a good supply of dried sage leaves for the winter months when my plants may be covered in a blanket of snow! If you don't grow sage, you can purchase fresh sage in the produce section of your grocery, or even dried sage in bulk or tea bags at your local health food store.

Sage may be my go-to sore throat remedy, but this rather pungent, gray-green perennial has much more to share! It has been called "the woman's herb" for several reasons. Sage has the ability to help with irregular menses. It can increase blood flow in cases of amenorrhea (scanty periods) or regulate bleeding with dysmenorrhea (painful, heavy periods). Sage tea can even help mammary glands stop milk production when a mom has weaned her baby.

Sage helps alleviate some of the discomforts of menopause, as well. As a sudorific herb, it helps with excessive sweating and those "tropical" moments, e.g. night sweats or hot flashes. In these cases, brew the tea, strain, it and then drink it room temperature or cool.

For best results in of all of these situations, a therapeutic dose is needed. One cup of sage tea is not enough. I always suggest using a 1 quart glass canning jar with a good lid. The recipe above makes enough for one day, which would be 3-4 cups of tea. The therapeutic dose is a minimum of 3 cups of the herbal tea. This has a wonderful healing effect on the body.

Sage is much more than tasty turkey stuffing! Remember sage and try it next time that you're in need!

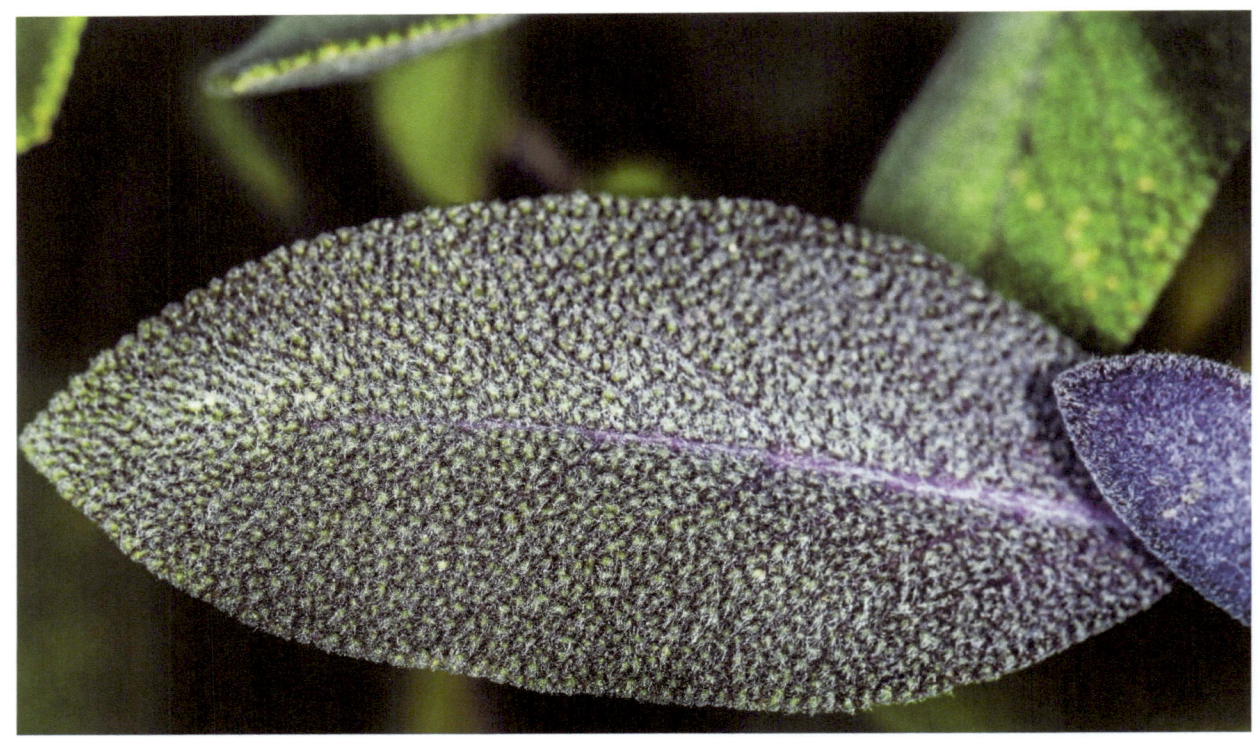

Sage History and Mythology

Heather Lanham

Why should a man die whilst sage grows in his garden?

~ *Ancient Proverb*

Sage may be an herb known over the entire planet. Some form grows in every populated country on our planet. Its Latin name, *salvia* means "to be saved" and it has been spoken of as *S. Salvatrix*, or Sage the Savior. One of my favorite types of sage is clary sage. There is not much that could be better in my world, unless it were perhaps camphor when I have a stuffy nose!

Darling sage has been well loved by the French. In one district it was supposed that sage aided with grief of the body and the mind, and in a few places it was customary to sow the graves with it. A French couplet about sage reads, "Sage helps the nerves and by its powerful might Palsy is cured and fever put into flight." Garden clary sage was known in France as *Toute-Bonne* due to it medicinal value.

In Mexico there is a variety known by another name entirely. Though chia seeds are quite well known, I doubt very many know that this sweet little mucilaginous seed so famed for little growing statues or used so widely as part of a healthy diet are, in fact, a variety of sage. The Latin name for chia is *Salvia Hispanica*. I have eaten chia as a kind of pudding, and it was a most odd sensation. To me, it was a bit like how I imagine eating caviar would be.

The English have their own love of sage and their own proverbs regarding it. It is said, "He that would live for aye, Must eat sage in May." I wonder if perhaps sage had certain qualities only realized in May during the time that this proverb was created? John Gerard mentions sage in 1597 as being well known to English gardens, with several varieties growing in his own. Some believed sage leaves should be munched on for 9 consecutive mornings while fasting as a cure for ague.

Italian peasants ate sage as a preserver of health, while in many other places it was eaten with bread and butter. Many times it has been said there is no more wholesome way to eat it. There is a certain species common to Greece called *Salvia Pomifera*, or applebearing sage. This sage grows fleshy protuberances that are called sage apples due to the punctures of a particular wasp. They were found in the markets after being candied and became a sort of sweetmeat, which was a great delicacy once upon a time.

There was also an Arab belief that, if your sage grew well, you would live a long time. Hungarian gypsies used sage to attract good and repel evil.

Sage is also part of the tale of the flight of Mary, Joseph, and the babe Jesus in some circles.

The flight into Egypt
and the miracles:
The Legend of the Sage plant

By Joseph Roumanille

Retold by M. Toussaint-Samat

"While the savage and bloodthirsty butchers of King Herod scoured the countryside around Bethlehem, cutting the throats of little children, Mary fled through the mountains of Judea, clutching her new-born tightly against her trembling heart. Seeing a village, Joseph ran ahead to ask for hospitality or even just a little water to bathe the little one. Alas, the nature of the people of this sad country was such that no one was prepared to offer anything, not water, shelter, not even a kind word.

Now while the poor mother was alone, seated by the side of the road nursing the child, her husband took the donkey to drink from a communal well. What did she hear but shouts getting closer as the ground shook under the hooves of approaching horses.

Herod's soldiers!

Where to hide? Not the slightest cave nor the smallest palm tree was to be seen. The only thing close to Mary was a bush where a rose was beginning to bloom.

'Rose, beautiful rose, begged the poor mother, open out all your petals and hide this infant whom they want to kill and his half-dead mother.'

The rose, wrinkling the pointed button which served as its nose, replied:

'Get on your way quickly, young woman, because the butchers could brush by me and blemish me. Go see the clove close by. Tell her to shelter you. She has enough flowers to conceal you.'

'Clove, pretty clove, begged the fugitive, spread out so that your mass will hide this child condemned to death and his exhausted mother.'

The clove shook the little heads of her flowers and refused without even explaining why:

'On your way, you poor wretch. I don't even have time to listen to you. I am too busy putting out blooms all over. Go see the sage plant close by. She has nothing better to do than dispense charity.'

'Ah! Sage, good sage, begged the unhappy woman, spread your leaves to hide this innocent whose life is in such danger and his mother who is half-dead with hunger, fatigue and fear.'

The sage plant then blossomed so abundantly that it covered all the earth and its velvety leaves created a canopy under which the God-child and His mother sheltered. On the road, the butchers passed by without seeing a thing. At the sound of their steps, Mary shivered in terror but the baby, caressed by the leaves, smiled. Then, as suddenly as they had come, the soldiers were gone.

When they had gone, Mary and Jesus came out from their green and flower-bedecked refuge. 'Sage, holy sage, many thanks. I bless you for your good deed which everyone will henceforth remember.'

When Joseph found them, he had a hard time keeping up with the donkey, which had been restored by a huge plateful of barley that a decent man had given him.

Mary remounted the animal, hugging her saved child to her. And Michael, the Archangel of God, descended from the realms of Heaven to keep them company and show them the shortest way they could journey in easy stages to Egypt."

References

- www.botanical.com/botanical/mgmh/s/sages-05.html
- www.avogel.ch/en/plant-encyclopaedia/salvia_officinalis.php
- www.trilliumfloral.com/Wedding-Legends.htm
- http://peninsulalighthouse.wordpress.com/2012/11/24/plant-lore-luck-flower-to-yule-log/
- http://www.indianmirror.com/ayurveda/sage.html
- http://www.culture.gouv.fr/culture/noel/angl/sauge.htm

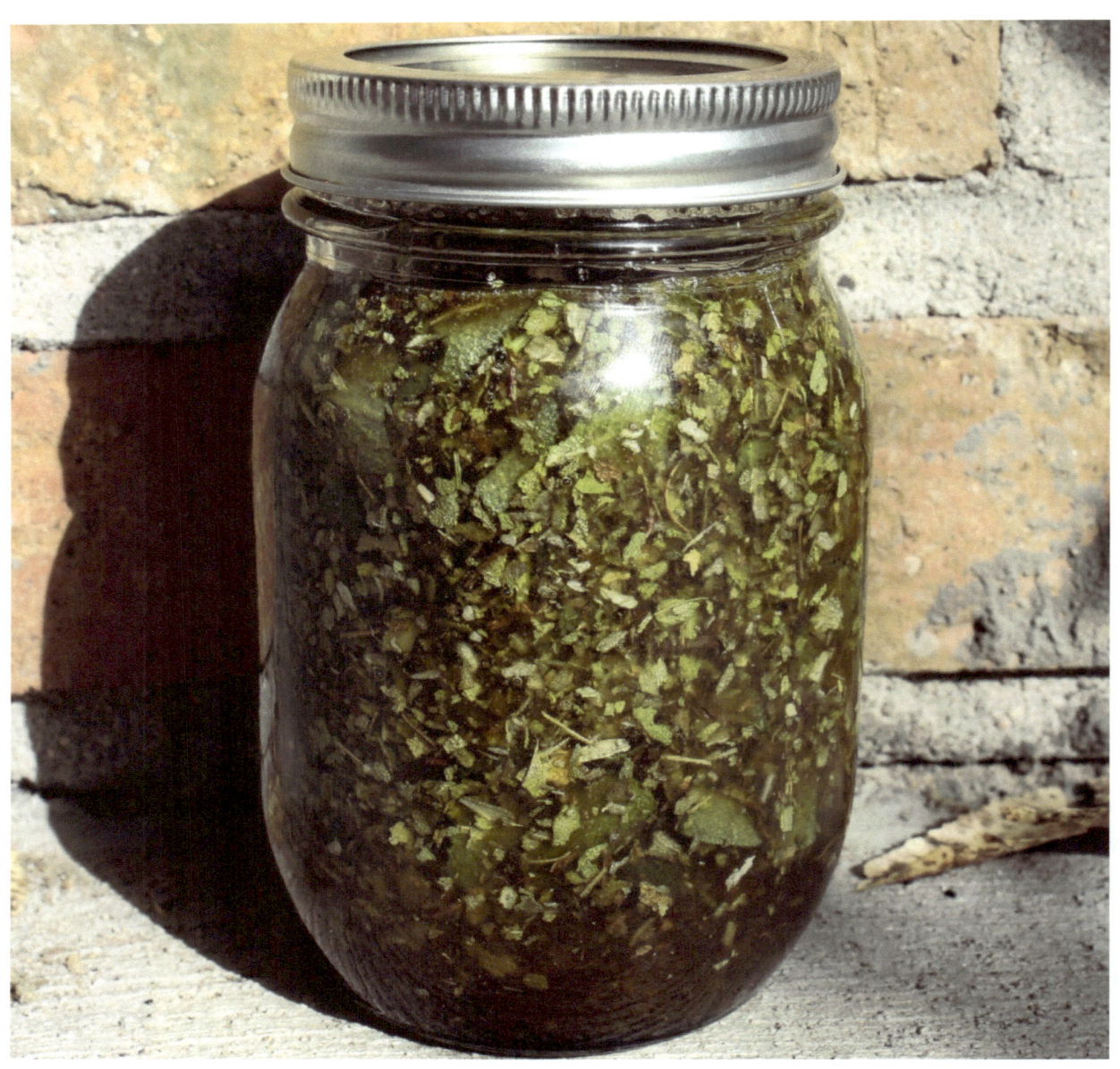

Sage and Oxymel Honey

Jan Berry

Sage is a wonderful ally to have on hand for cold and flu season. Using just a few simple ingredients from your kitchen, you can make the following two home remedies that are excellent treatments for coughs, sore throats, and congestion.

NOTE: These recipes are not intended for use by pregnant or nursing women.

Honey & Sage Sore Throat and Cough Syrup

Ingredients

- sage leaves, fresh

- raw honey

Directions

Add whole fresh sage leaves to a jar until it's ¼ to ½ full. Pour raw honey over the leaves until the jar is full. Stir with a chopstick or table knife to release any air pockets, then top off with more honey if needed.

Cover the jar and store in a cool, dark place for around a week or two. After this time, spoon or strain out the leaves. You'll be left with a sage infused honey syrup. Take by the spoonful for sore throats, colds, and coughs as needed.

Sage Oxymel

An oxymel is another name for a sweet and sour syrup. It's made by infusing herb(s) in both vinegar and honey and is oftentimes used to treat respiratory issues. I like to combine sage with other herbs such as rosemary and thyme when making an oxymel, but you can use sage by itself as well.

Ingredients

- sage leaves, fresh or dried

- optional, herb mix of choice, fresh or dried

- raw honey

- apple cider vinegar

Directions

First, fill a small jar about ½ to ¾ full of herbs. Use more for fresh herbs, less for dried.

Pour raw honey till the herbs are covered, then fill the remainder of the jar with apple cider vinegar. The ratio of honey to vinegar depends a lot on the desired taste you'd like. For a sweeter oxymel, use equal amounts of honey and vinegar. For a more sour taste, fill the jar about 1/3 full of honey and 2/3 with vinegar. Don't get hung up on precise amounts; since both vinegar and honey are natural preservatives, you can't mess up the mixture by altering ratios.

Use a chopstick or table knife to stir the mixture and remove any air bubbles. Cover with a plastic lid, or a piece of plastic wrap between a metal lid and jar. If you don't take this step, the acid in the vinegar will corrode metal over time, causing an unpleasant taste that will ruin your oxymel.

Let the herbs infuse for about two weeks, shaking occasionally. After that time has passed, strain out the plant material and store your finished oxymel in a sterile jar. I like to keep mine in the refrigerator or other very cool, dark place. Shelf life is at least one year.

Take by the spoonful as needed for sore throats, thick congested coughs, or as a general treatment to combat cold and respiratory symptoms.

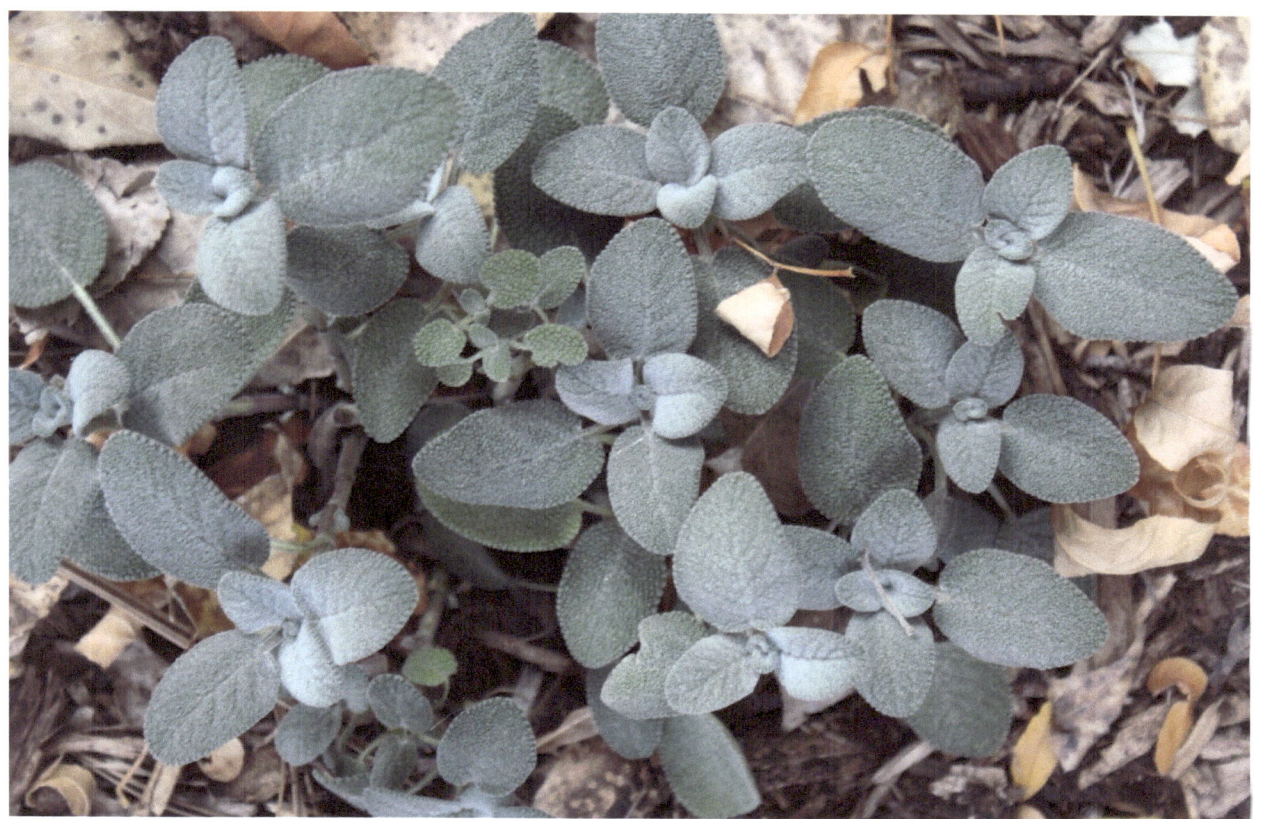

Sage for the Digestion and General Regulation of "Fluxes"

Nina Katz

As the nineteenth-century herbals put it, sage helps stop "fluxes," i.e. any excessive flow in the body, or excessively liquid flow. For example, nursing mothers use sage when they want to decrease the milk supply. As a drying remedy, sage is excellent in the treatment of diarrhea. Sage can be a fairly radical treatment, so be careful not to use too much. If you use it to treat IBS or IBD with a tendency to oscillate between the two extremes, use only a small amount so as not to cause too dramatic a shift. A simple short infusion of a quarter of a teaspoon will usually suffice. Another option is to combine sage with a gentler remedy, such as spearmint. A teaspoon of spearmint with a pinch of sage would make a mild but effective tea for getting the guts back on track.

Interestingly, sage doesn't only stop excessive flow, but it can also help to balance fluids, specifically in people with dry constitutions. Someone who tends to run dry, perhaps a Vata in the Ayurvedic classification, someone with dry skin and dry eyes, or other symptoms of dryness, may benefit from sage. For Vata or otherwise constitutionally dry people, sage tweaks the balance, so that instead of dryness or oscillation, all the fluxes shift slowly and subtly into harmony. It is especially appropriate for constitutionally dry or Vata types with digestive problems, such as chronic gastritis, IBS, or Ulcerative Colitis.

Because it can be so dramatically drying, using it as a culinary herb can also be an effective treatment. Of course, you can always balance it with soothing, moistening herbs and foods such as sassafras or okra to mitigate its effects, or simply use a small pinch in a large dish. If you're planning to include sage in your Thanksgiving menu, do it with awareness and balance so that your guests avoid the typical post-feast bellyache. Adding some general digestive herbs, such as ginger, will help too, as will a salad with some bitter greens, such as dandelion or arugula. A special bitters beverage will help as well, of course, and earn you accolades from grateful guests who go home feeling surprisingly comfortable.

Bitters

Ingredients

- 1 C dandelion root
- 2-3 in ginger root
- 2 qt water
- handful of spearmint
- optional, sage
- maple syrup

Directions

Decoct dandelion and ginger root in water for at least half an hour. Turn off the heat and add a handful of spearmint. If the indications are right, add a pinch or two of sage. You can also substitute a pinch of sage for the spearmint. Steep for an extra ten minutes, then strain and add a generous dollop of maple syrup. Serve neat, or add a splash to the beverage of your choice.

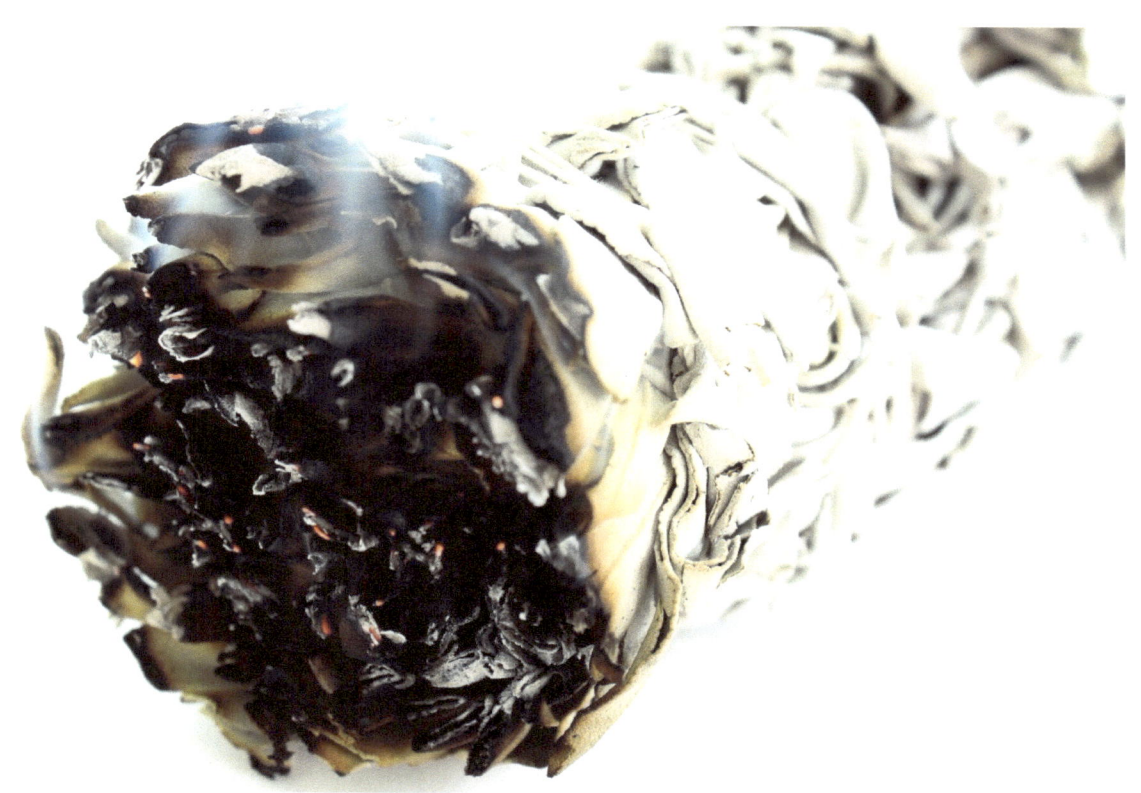

Sage Spirit Medicine

Balance of the Spiritual and Mundane
& Commitment to the Soul Journey

Darcey Blue

Dearest sage, an ally for our bodies, minds, and spirits. Her name, *Salvia*, is derived from the Latin, *Salvere*, to save or be well. In how many ways does she save us? Garden sage is one of our most multifaceted and versatile herbal allies, affecting the digestive, circulatory, nervous, and mucous membrane tissues and systems. Not only is garden sage a storehouse of medicine, but we have numerous other fragrant *Salvia* species available to us in our cultivated and wild gardens that we know and love well.

- Clary sage (*S. sclarea*) and her sweet scent that uplifts spirits and balances women's bodies.
- White sage (*S. apiana*), burned as a sacred smudge to clear heavy energy.
- Chia sage (*S. hispanica* or *S. columbariae*) for its nutritious and demulcent seeds.

- Red Sage/Tan Shen/Danshen (*S. miltiorrhiza*), used in Traditional Chinese Herbalism to move blood, stagnation, and heat.
- Diviners Sage (*S. divinorum*), and its controversial psychotropic entheogenic properties.

Though is it clear that all sages vary somewhat in their most prominent medicinal uses, there are some common threads that sage – from garden sage to white sage and beyond – can become our spiritual plant allies. As with any plant ally, I encourage you to take your own personal plant ally journey to discover what the plant has to say to you, especially if you have a particular favorite sage species to work with. It may have special and unique gifts to offer you in addition to what I have to share. Here is a short, guided meditation to help you take a little journey to visit with sage. [Guided Journey to Sage](#)

Sage is most well known as a spiritual plant ally for smudging. During smudging the dried leaves are burned either in a bundle or loose over a coal to create a thick, fragrant smoke that is used to clear the energy in a room, to create and invite sacred space, and to remove heavy or toxic energy on a person's physical or energetic body. But why sage? It's not just because of the nice smell; sage is an ally that specifically helps us align with higher spiritual energies and commit to our higher wisdom of the soul, even in the face of worldly temptations.

There are often times in life when we have an intuitive knowing or conscious understanding of what is in our best and highest interest as a spiritual human on our journey, regardless of what spiritual path or truth you follow. It is also true that life continually places opportunities in front of us to choose our actions that keep us in alignment with our higher purpose, by tempting us with things that may stray us from our course. You know the game; there is that tempting relationship that would inevitably become a distraction or toxic interference in your life, or the choice to take one job over another. One job may tempt with higher pay, but takes us further from our personal alignment and purpose.

When we need to find clarity on those choices, it is this medicine that sage offers. When we need support to stay the course. When we are tempted by our emotional or physical vices and need a friend to steer us right. Sage. Burn the sage and smudge your heart and your hands, your feet and your head. Get grounded in your spiritual and personal truth, not momentary distraction or tempting lures. Oftentimes when I am faced with such situations, my emotions are high, bordering on anxiety, desperation, or fear. A smudge and deep breathing can help me move through those moments with more grace. A dropperful of sage tincture can have a similar effect, and I like to keep a bottle of sage elixir on hand for such purposes. Garden, white, or black sage are wonderful for this.

Sage is also that ally to help us find and maintain balance in our lives between our worldly mundane duties and activities – like cleaning the dishes, running the kids to school, and paying the bills – and our need for regular, spiritual practices and activities which nourish our soul and spirit – like a daily yoga or meditation practice, connection with our spiritual guides and allies, time spent in nature, and visits to our spiritual communities.

Sage can teach us about finding that balance in our world in small yet meaningful ways. Oftentimes we do not maintain a daily practice for our spirits because we feel it has to take a lot of time or energy. Setting aside a whole hour for meditation and yoga can feel daunting, especially if your life is very full and busy. This is all the more reason to carve out a little space for your spirit. A simple five minute sit in the garden with a bit of sage burning can ground us in the Earth and her abundance of energy, and is sometimes all the medicine we need to begin with. Let sage help you create moments of spiritual balance and well being.

And, last but not least, sage is the ally to help us with our daily energetic hygiene. Does it strike you as odd that we shower and brush our teeth every day in order to keep our bodies clean and healthy, but we don't always perform daily spiritual and energetic hygiene practices? Why don't we keep our energy bodies as clean as our physical bodies? I often enjoy making an energetic clearing tea blend with white sage, peppermint, and rose to sip when I need to do some emotional clearing. A daily practice of smudging with dried sage or brushing the skin with fresh sage (and rosemary and lavender too) keeps our energetic, spiritual, and emotional bodies clear of the heavy and parasitic energies that tend to get attracted to weak boundaries. It allows us to call on a sacred space, spiritual allies, and our higher selves for a few moments on conscious intention to be whole and aligned, and to shed heavy energy in our thoughts.

So, whether your garden is growing common garden sage, or you have wild and fragrant white or black sage in your mountains, or you plant a beautiful pineapple or clary sage in a pot on your patio, allow the spiritual medicine of sage to guide you into balance, alignment, sacred space, and awareness in your life.

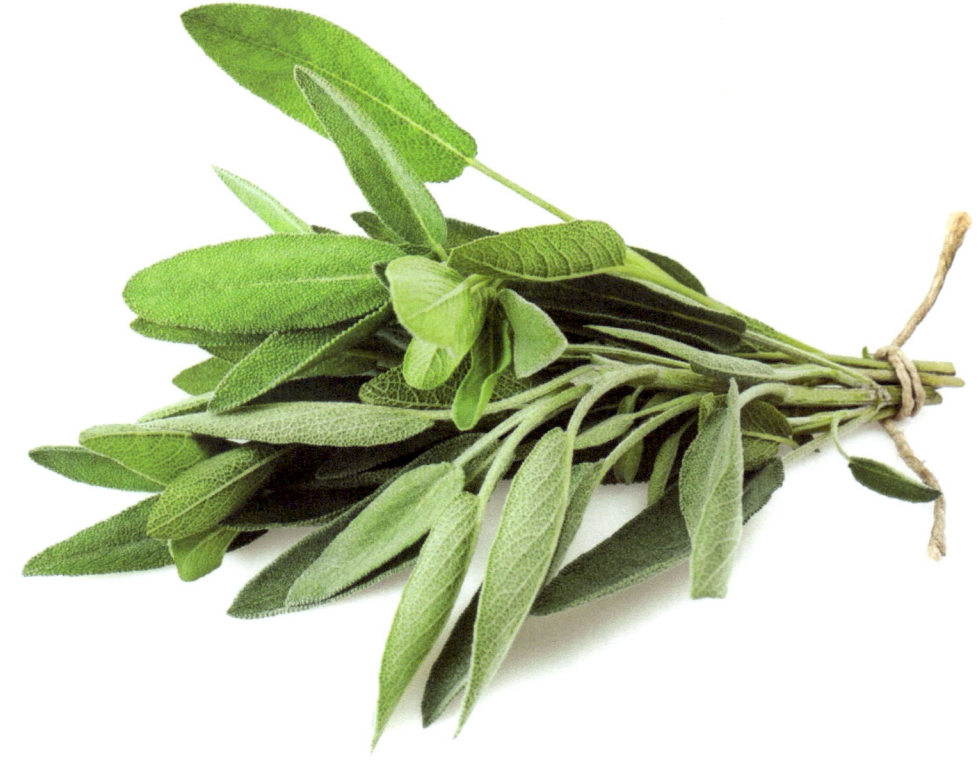

A Glossary of Herbalism

Nina Katz

Do you feel befuddled by all of those terms? Are you curious about what a menstruum might be, or a nervine? Wondering what the exact difference is between an infusion and a decoction? Or what it means to macerate? Read on; the herbalist lexicographer will reveal it all!

Ad*ap*togen	n.	An herb that enhances one's ability to thrive despite stress. Eleuthero, or Siberian Ginseng *(Eleutherococcus senticosus)* is a well-known adaptogen.
A*e*rial *parts*	n. pl.	The parts of a plant that grow above ground. Stems, leaves, and flowers are all aerial parts, in contrast to roots and rhizomes.
A*l*terative	n.	An herb that restores the body to health gradually and sustainably by strengthening one or more of the body's systems, such as the digestive or lymphatic system, or one or more of the vital organs, such as the liver or kidneys. Burdock *(Arctium lappa)* is an alternative.
	adj.	Restoring health gradually, as by strengthening one or more of the body's systems or vital organs.
Anthel*min*tic	n.	A substance that eliminates intestinal worms.
Anthel*min*	adj.	Being of or concerning a substance that eliminates intestinal worms.
Anti-ca*tarr*hal	n.	A substance that reduces or slows down the production of phlegm.
	adj.	Being of or concerning a substance that reduces or slows down the production of phlegm.
Anti-emetic	n.	A substance that treats nausea. Ginger *(Zingiber officinale)* is anti-emetic.
	adj.	Being of or concerning a substance that treats nausea.
Anti-mi*cro*bial	n.	An herb or a preparation that helps the body fight off microbial infections, whether viral, bacterial, fungal, or parasitic. Herbal anti-microbials may do this by killing the microbes directly, but more often achieve this by enhancing immune function and helping the body to fight off disease and restore

		balance.
	adj.	Being of or concerning an herb or a preparation that helps the body fight off microbial infections.
Aperient	n.	A gentle laxative, such as seaweed, plantain seeds *(Plantago spp.)*, or ripe bananas.
	adj.	Being of or concerning a gentle laxative.
Aphrodisiac	n.	A substance that enhances sexual interest or desire.
	adj.	Being of or relating to a substance that enhances sexual interest or desire.
Astringent	n.	A food, herb, or preparation that causes tissues to constrict, or draw in. Astringents help stop bleeding, diarrhea, and other conditions in which some bodily substance is flowing excessively. Some astringents, such as Wild Plantain *(Plantago major)*, draw so powerfully that they can remove splinters.
	adj	Causing tissues to constrict, and thereby helping to stop excessive loss of body fluids.
Bitter	n.	A food, herb, or preparation that stimulates the liver and digestive organs through its bitter flavor. Dandelion *(Taraxacum officinale)* and Gentian *(Gentiana lutea)* are both bitters. Also called *digestive bitter.*
Carminative	n.	A food, herb, or preparation that reduces the buildup or facilitates the release of intestinal gases. Cardamom *(Amomum spp. and Elettaria spp)* and Fennel *(Foeniculum vulgare)* are carminatives.
	adj.	Characterized as reducing the buildup or facilitating the release of intestinal gases.
Carrier Oil	n.	A non-medicinal oil, such as olive or sesame oil, used to dilute an essential oil.
Catarrh	n.	An inflammation of the mucous membranes resulting in an overproduction of phlegm.
Compound	v.	To create a medicinal formula using two or more components.
	n.	An herbal preparation consisting of two or more herbs.

*Com*press	n.	A topical preparation consisting of a cloth soaked in a liquid herbal extract, such as an infusion or decoction, and applied, usually warm or hot, to the body. A washcloth soaked in a hot ginger decoction and applied to a sore muscle is a compress.
De*coct*	v.	To prepare by simmering in water, usually for at least 20 minutes. One usually decocts barks, roots, *rhizomes*, hard seeds, twigs, and nuts.
De*coct*ion	n.	An herbal preparation made by simmering the plant parts in water, usually for at least 20 minutes.
De*mul*cent	n.	An herb with a smooth, slippery texture soothing to the mucous membranes, i.e. the tissues lining the respiratory and digestive tracts. Slippery elm *(Ulmus rubra)*, marshmallow root *(Althaea officinalis)*, and sassafras *(Sassafras albidum, Sassafras officinale)* are all demulcents.
	adj.	Having a smooth, slippery texture that soothes the mucous membranes.
Diapho*ret*ic	n.	An herb or preparation that opens the pores of the skin, facilitates sweat, and thereby lowers fevers. In Chinese medicine, diaphoretics are said to "release the exterior."□ Yarrow *(Achillea millefolium)* is a diaphoretic.
	adj.	Opening the pores, facilitating sweat, and thereby lowering fevers.
Di*ges*tive	n.	An herb, food, or preparation that promotes the healthy breakdown, assimilation, and elimination of food, as by gently stimulating the digestive tract in preparation for a meal. Dandelion *(Taraxacum officinale)* and bitter salad greens are digestives.
	adj. 1	Concerning or being part of the bodily system responsible for the breakdown, assimilation, and elimination of food.
	adj. 2	Promoting the healthy breakdown, assimilation, and/or elimination of food.
Diu*ret*ic	n.	A substance that facilitates or increases urination. Diuretics can improve kidney function and treat swelling. Excessive use of diuretics can also tax the

		kidneys. Stinging Nettles *(Urtica dioica)*, cucumbers, and coffee are all diuretics.
	adj.	Facilitating or increasing urination.
Em*men*agogue	n.	An herb or preparation that facilitates or increases menstrual flow. Black cohosh *(Cimicifuga racemosa)* is an emmenagogue. Emmenagogues are generally contraindicated in pregnancy.
	adj.	Facilitating or increasing menstrual flow.
Es*sen*tial *Oil*	n.	An oil characterized by a strong aroma, strong taste, the presence of terpines, and by vaporizing in low temperatures. Essential oils are components of many plants, and when isolated, make fairly strong medicine used primarily externally or for inhalation, and usually not safe for internal use.
	n. 1	A preparation made by chemically removing the soluble parts of a substance into a solvent or menstruum. Herbalists often make extracts using water, alcohol, glycerin, vinegar, oil, or combinations of these. Infusions, medicinal vinegars, tinctures, decoctions, and medicinal oils are all extracts.
	n. 2	A tincture.
Ex*tract*	v.	To remove the soluble parts of a substance into a solvent or menstruum by chemical means.
Febrifuge	n.	An herb or preparation that lowers fevers. Yarrow *(Achillea millefolium)*, ginger *(Zingiber officinale)*, and boneset *(Eupatorium perfoliatum)* are all febrifuges.
Ga*lac*tagogue	n.	A substance that increases the production or flow of milk; a remedy that aids lactation. Nettle *(Urtica dioica)* and hops *(Humulus lupulus)* are galactagogues.
*Glan*dular	n.	A substance that treats the adrenal, thyroid, or other glands. Nettle seeds *(Urtica dioica)* are a glandular for the adrenals.
	adj.	Relating to or treating the adrenal, thyroid, or other glands.
He*pat*ic	n.	A substance that treats the liver. Dandelion *(Taraxacum officinale)* is a hepatic.
Hyp*not*ic	n.	An herb or preparation that induces sleep. Chamomile *(Matricaria recutita)* and valerian *(Valeriana officinale)* are both hypnotics.

	adj.	Inducing sleep.
Infuse	v.	To prepare by steeping in water, especially hot water, straining, and squeezing the marc.
Infusion	n.	A preparation made by first steeping one or more plants or plant parts in water, most often hot water, and then straining the plant material, usually while squeezing the marc. An infusion extracts the flavor, aroma, and water-soluble nutritional and medicinal constituents into the water.
Long Infusion	n.	An infusion that steeps for three or more hours. Long infusions often steep overnight.
Lymphatic	n.	A substance that stimulates the circulation of lymph or *tonifies* the vessels or organs involved in the circulation or storage of lymph.
Macerate	v.	To soak a plant or plant parts in a *menstruum* so as to extract the medicinal constituents chemically.
Marc	n.	The plant material left after straining a preparation made by steeping, simmering, or macerating.
Menstruum	n.	*(Plural, **menstrua** or **menstruums**.)* The solvent used to extract the medicinal and/or nutritional constituents from a plant. Water, alcohol, vinegar, and glycerin are among the more common menstrua.
Mucilage	n.	A thick, slippery, *demulcent* substance produced by a plant or microorganism.
Mucilaginous	n.	Having or producing mucilage; *demulcent.* Okra, marshmallow root *(Althaea officinalis)*, sassafras *(Sassafras albidum, Sassafras officinale)*, and slippery elm *(Ulmus rubra)* are all mucilaginous.
Nervine	n.	An herb or preparation that helps with problems traditionally associated with the nerves, such as mental health issues, insomnia, and pain.
	adj.	Helping with problems traditionally associated with the nerves, such as mental health issues, insomnia, and pain.
Pectoral	n.	A substance that treats the lungs or the respiratory system.
Poultice	n.	A mass of plant material or other substances, usually mashed, gnashed, moistened, or heated, and placed directly on the skin. Sometimes covered by a cloth or adhesive. A plantain *(Plantago spp.)* poultice can draw splinters out.

Rhizome	n.	A usually horizontal stem that grows underground, is marked by nodes from which roots grow down, and branches out to produce a network of new plants growing up from the nodes.
Salve	[sæv] n.	A soothing ointment prepared from beeswax combined with oil, usually medicinal oil, and used in topical applications.
Short Infusion	n.	An *infusion* that steeps for a relatively short period of time, usually 5-30 minutes.
Sedative	n.	A substance that calms and facilitates sleep. Valerian *(Valeriana officinale)* is a sedative.
Sedative	adj.	Calming and facilitating sleep.
*Sim*ple	n.	An herbal preparation, such as a tincture or decoction, made from one herb alone.
*Sim*pler	n.	An herbalist who prepares and recommends primarily *simples* rather than compounds.
Spp.	abbr. n.pl.	Species. *Used to indicate more than one species in the same botanical family. Echinacea spp.* includes both *Echinacea purpurea* and *Echinacea angustifolium*, among other species. *Plantago spp.* includes both *Plantago major* and *Plantago lanceolata.*
*Stim*ulant	n.	An herb or preparation that increases the activity level in an organ or body system. Echinacea *(Echinacea spp.)* is an immunostimulant; it stimulates the immune system. Cayenne *(Capsicum spp.)* is a circulatory stimulant. Rosemary is a stimulant to the nervous, digestive, and circulatory systems.
*Sudo*rific	adj.	Increasing sweat or facilitating the release of sweat; cf. *diaphoretic.*
Syrup	n.	A sweet liquid preparation, often made by adding honey or sugar to a decoction.
Tea	n.	A drink made by steeping a plant or plant parts, especially *Camellia sinensis.*
Tisane	n.	An herbal beverage made by decoction or short infusion and not prepared from the tea plant

		(Camellia sinensis).
*Tin*cture	n.	A preparation made by macerating one or more plants or plant parts in a *menstruum,* usually alcohol or glycerin, straining, and squeezing the *marc* in order to extract the chemical constituents into the *menstruum.*
	v.	To prepare by *macerating* in a *menstruum,* straining, and squeezing the marc in order to extract the chemical constituents.
Tonic	n.	A substance that strengthens one or more organs or systems, or the entire organism. Stinging nettle *(Urtica dioica)* is a general tonic, as well as a specific kidney, liver, and hair tonic. Red raspberry leaf *(Rubus idaeus)* is a reproductive tonic; Mullein *(Verbascum thapsus)* is a respiratory tonic.
*Ton*ify	v.	To strengthen. Nettle *(Urtica dioica)* tonifies the entire body.
Vola*tile* Oil	n.	An oil characterized by volatility, or rapid vaporization at relatively low temperatures; c*f*. *essential oil.*
Vulnerary	n.	A substance that soothes and heals wounds. Comfrey *(Symphytum officinale)* is an excellent vulnerary.
	adj.	Being or concerning a substance that soothes and heals wounds.

Disclaimer

Nothing provided by Natural Living Mamma LLC, Natural Herbal Living Magazine, or Herb Box should be considered medical advice. Nothing included here is approved by the FDA and the information provided herein is for informational purposes only. Always consult a botanically knowledgeable medical practitioner before starting any course of treatment, especially if you are pregnant, breastfeeding, on any medications, or have any health problems. Natural Living Mamma LLC is not liable for any action or inaction you take based on the information provided here.